Acknowledgement

The inspiration for this book came from
the monthly columns I wrote for
The DO magazine
published by the American Osteopathic Association
and re-published in an anthology of columns
Effective Medical Communication.
I have borrowed heavily from those columns and
I express my deep appreciation for permission to do so.

For more detailed information about any of these
subjects, please consult the book
Effective Medical Communication

Other books by the author

Pediatrics: Some Uncommon Views on Some Common Problems

Professionally Speaking: Public Speaking for Health Professionals

Oratoria Para Professionales de la Salud

Medical Writing 101: A Primer for Health Professionals

Parenthood: Laugh and Understand Your Child

Ethical Problems in Pediatrics: A Dozen Dilemmas

Effective Medical Communication: An Anthology of Columns

Looking Back . . . at SECOM

PRACTICING FOR PRACTICE

A handbook for residents about to enter practice (especially for those in Internal Medicine, Family Medicine, Pediatrics and Obstetrics-Gynecology) with emphasis on patient care

Arnold Melnick, DO, MSc, DHL (Hon.), FACOP

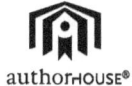
authorHOUSE®

AuthorHouse™
1663 Liberty Drive
Bloomington, IN 47403
www.authorhouse.com
Phone: 1-800-839-8640

© 2012 by Arnold Melnick, DO, MSc, DHL(Hon), FACOP. All rights reserved.

No part of this book may be reproduced, stored in a retrieval system, or transmitted by any means without the written permission of the author.

Published by AuthorHouse   07/19/2012

ISBN: 978-1-4772-4038-0 (sc)
ISBN: 978-1-4772-4037-3 (e)

Library of Congress Control Number: 2012912278

Any people depicted in stock imagery provided by Thinkstock are models, and such images are being used for illustrative purposes only. Certain stock imagery © Thinkstock.

This book is printed on acid-free paper.

Because of the dynamic nature of the Internet, any web addresses or links contained in this book may have changed since publication and may no longer be valid. The views expressed in this work are solely those of the author and do not necessarily reflect the views of the publisher, and the publisher hereby disclaims any responsibility for them.

Contents

Dedication.. vii

Preface ix

Introduction... xi

Part One: Choosing a Potential Practice

First, A Look at the Scene You'll be Entering......3

Patients' Views 8

A U-turn 11

Your Practice Site 12

What Type of Practice for You? 17

Who Will Be Your Patients?
    And What Will They Bring? 21

Part Two: The Interpersonal Relationships

Your Office 27

Your Writings 43

Dedication

I dedicate this book to my dear friend, my internist
and my medical guru for fifty years

A. Alvin Greber, DO
Executive Dean for Professional Affairs
Health Professions Division
Nova Southeastern University

who has trained or help train hundreds of students,
interns and residents and who reviewed this
manuscript and made some pertinent suggestions

Preface

You are on the threshold of entering medical practice. Congratulations! You have been anticipating this great moment for some time.

Halt! Before you even start to look around, it is urgent that you pay attention to a number of things —considerations that are as important as, or more important than, which office space to rent or which group to join. For, you see, you are not applying for a summer job, or something to do short-term. You are about to make a life-long decision, which can become complicated unless you do a lot of advance thinking.

It involves a lot of introspection, some of which you may have already done. Where you would like to practice. Which hospital(s) you might want to be near. What kind of patients you want. How you want to be viewed by your patients. And so on.

These items might seem superfluous at this moment, but let me assure you that they are absolute necessities if you want to have a long and enjoyable professional career. Missteps that occur (some accidental, some circumstantial and some by hurried choices) often take long times to remedy.

It is important to learn good habits early, then you won't have to spend time in unlearning the bad habits when you become busy.

Thus, by preparing properly, you will be **Practicing for Practice.**

Arnold Melnick, DO

So enjoy this book, take seriously its recommendations—and don't hesitate to consult with practitioners whom you highly respect and would like to emulate. Medicine is known for its ubiquitous mentoring of younger physicians by more senior physicians. And some day, you can help younger members of the profession as they come along.

Introduction

OK, so you have studied your Gray's, your Harrison's, your Cecil's and the like, and you sit nervously anticipating your going into practice. But what didn't those great texts teach you? And what exposure did you have to real *patient care?*

Arbitrarily, we can divide the act of seeing patients into two parts: medical diagnosis/treatment and patient care. You've probably already heard of, or encountered, "Gee, Doctor X is a very fine physician but you have to wait in his office for an hour for your appointment." Another frequent comment is "Dr. Y is such a great diagnostician but he hardly talks to you." Directly in those two oft-repeated quotes lies the factor of patient care, the act of treating patients as human beings, considering all aspects of the patient's life and environment and feelings and apprehensions, so as to make that patient as comfortable as possible in the doctor's office. Add to that, the primary goal of meeting patients needs or, whenever possible, their wants.

A couple of years back, the *Wall Street Journal* conducted a study with Harris Interactive, a polling company. Two findings had serious implications in the practice of medicine. First, it was found that patients placed more importance on the interpersonal skills of their doctors than they did on the medical experience, knowledge and proficiency of those physicians. And second, their statistical study established that patients have strong feelings about and desires to seek a new physician when skills in interpersonal activities are inadequate or unsatisfactory.

So, this book is an attempt to present some helpful hints for beginning a practice, and for the management of patients (not their illnesses)—based on a lifetime of pediatric office practice, extensive hospital experience and some years as a medical educator. Because this aspect is my theme, I will not deal with the organization or management or finances of practice or any business aspects—just the inter-personal relations with patients. I have deliberately avoided matters dealing with the business or mechanics of a practice. These are best left to practice management consultants, who have so much to contribute in these areas.

I hope I am successful in helping you, the reader, to find ways to become a successful medical practitioner who is also skilled in patient care. Either way, I wish you great success—and enjoyment—in your coming medical practice. From me to you: GOOD LUCK!

Part One

Choosing a Potential Practice

First, A Look at the Scene You'll be Entering

Going into practice, you'll be entering a "new" world, inhabited by thousands of fine physicians providing excellent medical services to a multitude of patients, and along with that, giving good patient care, the human side of practice.

This chapter is intended to expose you to the small minority of exceptions, the occasions of poor patient care, and of dissatisfied patients. My purpose is to try to help you avoid those kinds of practice problems.

First, just to orient you, let's look at some of the more positive kinds of practitioners. All are actual incidents.

Examples of the good practitioners
Personal contact

Dr. A entered the examining room, walked directly to the patient and, placing his hand gently on hers, asked, "Why do you think your family doctor wanted you to have a consultation with me?" Friendly, comforting, reassuring and letting the patient know he was interested in her views of her problems—and making a personal contact by touching her hand.

Showing concern

Dr. B came into the waiting room to get her next patient (no cold aides). She called the patient by name, took the patient into her consultation room, where they sat on either side of her desk. She took notes of what the patient said as they both spoke in an informal manner. When it came time for the examination, Dr. B escorted her to the examining room next door. An attitude of not rushing, and showing concern for the patient.

Orienting patients

Dr. C entered the room with another doctor, who was dressed in "whites," walked over to the examining table where the patient sat and said, "Good morning, Mr. Karp, would you mind if my resident, Dr. Smith, started your examination? I'll be back in a few minutes." The patient knew exactly what was going on. No strange doctor entering the room and starting to examine him. Smooth transition equals decreased patient anxiety. The same applies to any other personnel in the room (such as nurses, technicians) explaining what they do.

These examples are not meant to tell you how to handle your patients, but are fine examples of courteous and considerate management of patients. And episodes like this can be multiplied thousands of times by fine physicians.

Examples of the other side

Here are a few stories, unfortunately of the other kind—and again, all are true.

Mr. X visited a new dermatologist's office and was placed in an examining room. Shortly, the doctor entered and, after a few questions, began to examine the patient's skin. Mr. X, who was very sophisticated in medical affairs, quietly asked, "Aren't you going to wash your hands first?" Fuming, the doctor's response was, "Get out of here. I don't want you for a patient!"

and he left the room. No need for me to explain further.

Mrs. A needed surgery to remove a thymoma from her chest. Recommended was a highly skilled surgeon, chair of Chest Surgery at a major hospital. She saw him twice-only twice-once at the initial office consultation and again when discharged from the hospital. In effect (with only a few minor exceptions), all he ever said to her was, "We'll operate on Monday" and "Are you ready to go home?" Nothing in-between, no explanation, no information, no interpersonal action. Yes, he was a great cutter and sewer, but was he a true physician?

My wife was under the care of a neurologist. Every time we went to his office, there was a 60-90 minute wait. We became friendly and on a first-name basis. At our last visit (it was our choice to leave his practice), I asked if I might make a suggestion about the long wait everyone endured; I suggested that he hire a good practice management consultant who would straighten out his appointment schedule, and once it was worked out, the physician would be able to tell his wife just what time he would be home for dinner—and the patients would no longer have to wait inordinate lengths of time for their appointments. His reply, with a wave of the hand, was "Oh, just come in near the end of office hours and you won't have to wait so long." Absolutely no concern for the 30 or so patients sitting in his office for 60-90 minutes. No concern for their discomfort. No concern for their anxieties. The only important thing apparently was that he was important enough for all those people to wait. Let's see: 30 patients times 75 minutes (average) is almost 40 hours of time wasted.

Multiplying that by just 3 days a week, it's 120 wasted human hours—and he didn't care!

Mrs. D felt a lump in her breast and at once went to her surgeon. (This was reported in a Philadelphia newspaper.) Appropriately, he did an immediate biopsy. Mrs. D waited patiently for a call with the test result. Finally, on a Friday night it came. "Mrs. D, this is Dr. X. Your test came back and you have cancer. Come in Monday morning and we'll discuss it." Totally distraught, and on the verge of tears, she inquired, "But what will I do in the meantime?" His cold-hearted reply was. "I told you to come in Monday morning and we would discuss it. Remember, you're not the only patient I have." Cold, heartless, uncaring—maybe a good operating surgeon but not a compassionate doctor. Physicians should try not to give worrisome news too far in advance to avoid severe patient anxiety—and should be reassuring when giving that news.

Mrs. R went to see a physician for a consultation. As he walked into the room, he put up his hand and said, "Don't talk to me. Just answer my questions." Such arrogance: first, that without hearing the patient's problems, he could instantly come up with the correct diagnosis and treatment, and second, that he did not want to take any information from the patient. He knew all the answers and "knew" he knew them, so why bother being human with the patient and getting all the vital information! He evidently never heard of the sage words of the great Sir William Osler, MD: Listen, the patient is telling you the diagnosis.

Dr. G was an orthopedic surgeon. In his office hours, he saw pre-operative patients, post-operative check-ups and consultations. He told everyone of them to come to his office at 1 PM on Friday (or another day). When they arrived, they found a sign-in book that determined the order in which he took his patients. Those who came a little late (or were preceded by other patients) would have to wait until he saw the first ones (sometimes 30 of these) on the list. Fair? Considerate? His actions sent a message of his philosophy (maybe subconscious): *Those patients have nothing else to do, they don't mind. Only my time is important. Only my time is money. Let them wait. Besides, I'm loaded with so many patients that if I lose a few of the sore-heads, I won't miss them.*

Not all doctors behave like this and these physicians may not do this all the time. But these things occur frequently enough that patients become upset and talk about it.

The reality
These incidents—good and bad—are all actual ones, but I believe both kinds are repeated in some form multiple times by those doctors and mirrored thousands of times by doctors across the country. And all are illustrative.

I painted this situation with a broad brush, but this is what's out there. And I want to help you in advance to avoid those bad approaches and become proficient in your interpersonal skills with patients.

Patients' Views

Most of us grew up with the old aphorism "The customer is always right"—a truism that applies to most businesses and transactions. Of course, there are variations in interpretation but almost always leaning in favor of the customer.

After all, what is the primary purpose of almost every business and profession? No matter what products they sell or what services they provide, it is customer satisfaction, or client satisfaction—or for us, patient satisfaction. In effect, it is mostly the needs and wants of the patient as much as possible. Without "customer satisfaction," eventually there are no more customers, and no more business or profession. Sure, there are instances in which "customer satisfaction" would be contrary to laws or good practices—or in Medicine would be illegal, immoral or bad medical practice. But in denying such instances, there are approaches that often retain "customer satisfaction."

So, in practice, you want to provide the best possible medicine and also treat the patient with human care so that there will be as much satisfaction as possible.

What, then, do patients think about medical practice? In the *Wall Street Journal* article mentioned in the Preface, some interesting statistics came through:

> 85% of the survey believed that treating a patient with dignity and respect was an important attitude for physicians to exhibit.
>
> 84% of them felt that the ability to listen carefully to the patient and be easy to talk to were important attributes for physicians.
>
> 58% urged the importance of having a physician who has a lot of experience in treating similar patients.
> (Author's Comment: Note the big difference between the human characteristics and professional experience.)

The chairman of the Harris Poll commented on the results, "The startling numbers show that doctors' training and knowledge of new medical treatments are less important to many patients than their interpersonal skills—treating patients with respect, listening carefully and really caring."

A few years ago, a physician opening a "boutique" practice bought a full-page newspaper ad listing the obstacles that patients faced in other types of practice and guaranteeing not to allow them in his practice. Among other things, he noted:

> "Calling for an appointment means several days to a week unless it is an emergency.
>
> 'Waiting in a doctor's waiting room for long periods of time (sometimes an hour or more).

"Short time frame with the doctor (usually 10 to 15 minutes or less).

"Ability to address only the reason for the visit (earache, cut, etc) and no other issues.

"Inability to get through to talk to the doctor on the telephone.

"Getting an answering machine with long waits instead of being able to talk to an actual person."

I hope these illustrative examples of poor doctor-patient interactions will establish for you that dissatisfaction of patients with the interpersonal relationships of many doctors does exist, and my goal being to keep you from similar mistakes.

A U-turn

So far, this book has seemed to be mainly on the negative side. That is not meant to demean any individual or any group. It was merely, in case you weren't already aware, to acquaint you with some of the wrong approaches to patients that exist out there in the big, wide world.

You know: learn from bad examples.

From here on, we will approach the subject in a positive way, with many suggestions and ideas—all based on my experience, my interactions with a multitude of physicians, my contact with many other people and a lot of reading. That does not mean that these are the only ways to practice; there's no exclusivity. But, perhaps reading this book will suggest to you other positive approaches. Maybe it will give you food for thought before you enter practice.

Above all, and I am convinced of this, patient care—the interpersonal actions between patient and physician—is equally important as keen medical ability. Both are needed for competency in medical practice. Unfortunately, as I've pointed out, sometimes doctors believe that *only* medical skill is important.

From here on out, I will try to take the high road, with suggestions for establishing excellent interpersonal relations with your future patients. That, combined with your medical skills, will make you a splendid physician, skilled in good patient care.

Your Practice Site

Where should you practice? A difficult question with difficult answers. You should try not to leave it to chance.

Now—not years from now, or after you start a practice—now is the time to think deeply on what your desires are from practice. Then, search for your wishes.

What do you have to consider?

Field of practice.

Maybe you have already decided. Maybe you are in or finishing a specific residency. You will have already decided. If you are still a student, you may need to look around, weigh the pros and cons of family medicine and all the other specialties. If you easily reach a conclusion, great, that's it. If you have difficulty, speak to a practitioner in the field or fields you are thinking about. Arrange a sit-down conference with that person, not a fast, five-minute hallway talk. Explore all the avenues, all the things you may be interested in, all the questions you may have. Perhaps do the same with other doctors in the same field Then do the same for any other field you are considering. If you are married, or contemplating marriage, spend time going over your findings and feelings with your mate—he or she will have to survive with you, hopefully, for many years after you've decided.

Where do you want to live?

This is one of the two *most important questions* driving your life, whether you realize it or not. Living where you want to live (or not) can improve your professional life (or destroy it). Are you a city-person who needs things like big sports teams, theatres, universities, much activity? Would you be able to get along in a rural atmosphere? Or the reverse: Are you a country-person who likes quiet, neighborliness, no rush or bustle—would you be happy in a traffic-laden, noisy city atmosphere? These are just two examples of the kinds of choice you should make. Maybe your preferences lie in-between. Do you feel the need to practice near a major hospital center or would you rather work in a small—or medium-sized community hospital? All of these considerations should be reviewed so that you settle in a community of your choice or come as close as you can.

Family considerations

Happiness of your family (or future family) and satisfactory living situations should be probably the most important consideration. They will have to live with whatever you choose—so pick wisely. And you will be happier and your practice more fulfilling. Consider where your family (present or later) would be most content? Your wife? Where would you want your children to grow up? I strongly believe that this is a basic underlying and primary decision you must make. So remember, always consult with your spouse or future spouse (or children if you have any)—that's more important than the color of your furniture, or size of your desk or other considerations. You cannot really be a happy practitioner in any field if your family and home life are under stress.

Additional considerations.

Here are some other questions that you should take a stab at answering *before* you start to look at practice sites—or at least consider while you are looking:

Size of practice. Would you rather emulate that colleague who works long days (and sometimes nights) with little time off—either for helping people or because he feels the need for greater income? Or would you rather limit your practice (yes, it can be done and still be a compassionate physician) to a size that is reasonable to you (to give you greater freedom for your personal and marital life)? There are many successful—and good—physicians on both sides of the coin. It is a matter of personal choice.

Income. Some people in life want to make as much money as is humanly possible. Some people want only those earnings that are comfortable to their reaching a certain goal to live the life they covet. Or in-between? Whichever way one chooses is fine, provided you do not prostitute yourself in the process. Only you (and your spouse) can decide this question.

There are a number of different methods of compensation for doctors in various positions: salary, salary with incentives, bonuses, perquisites, profit-sharing and many compensation packages that combine all or some of these. Sometimes a plan can be confusing, so unless the package is a straight salary deal, it is wise to seek input from a knowledgeable source—your practice management consultant, your accountant or your attorney. And do it before you make any decisions.

As a generalization, I divide income into separate considerations depending on the source of the monies:

Straight salary. This may be illustrated by a position in which you work exclusively for a single employer, such as a doctor-employee of a partnership or a hospital or any other group. The advantage of this mode is that you are guaranteed (if you continue to work satisfactorily) a fixed or near-fixed amount, steady with rare fluctuations. The other side is that your income is limited to that salary and just working longer or harder will not increase your take-home pay. Remember that with salaried positions, the payer usually has some or much control over the way you practice. Some feel that this is a satisfactory arrangement since it allows them to have a comfortable income and to enjoy other things in life.

Solo practice. This source of income is the profit from your practice. The advantages: What you take home is a product of how hard you work and how you control expenses. Need more money? Work harder or longer—or cut your expenses. Your income is entirely dependent on what you continue to produce every day. And there is no "boss" to tell you how to practice. But it brings on additional practice responsibilities.

Third party practice employment. This may be working for an HMO or a hospital or other entity or joining a partnership. Your income here is usually a salary or a base salary plus extras (there are often incentives). The advantage: You usually know your hours and your approximate income. The disadvantage: You are not independent; the payer almost always has some control over what you do and how you do it. There are a variety of such positions and a variety of compensation plans. Always consider how well you work with others or with a group. Can you take orders? Can you accept criticism or evaluations? This is important in making a decision.

While I am not suggesting that these are hard-and-fast boundaries, the more you think about them and the more you find yourself leaning in one direction, the easier it will be to choose a practice site.

Once you've decided these major questions, you are ready to look around for practice possibilities.

Remember two things:

1. When there is a payer, you automatically give up some control over what you do and how you practice.
2. With financial considerations, unless you are finance-smart, it is best to consult with your practice management consultant, your accountant or your attorney for advice—before you sign any contracts.

What Type of Practice for You?

A practice is *not* a practice is *not* a practice is *not* a practice. I have chosen those words carefully to emphasize the fact that there are many varieties of practice. Some are easily defined but many are combinations of the major types of practice.

It is helpful for you to know which varieties of practice you prefer (or do not want), but it should not influence your decision too much—unless you have strong feelings either way.

There are various classifications of practice (with many internal variations), but here are some generally accepted kinds:

Solo

Practicing alone means that you have full responsibility for everything you do—practice, business, employment of aides, and everything else. You have complete independence of thought and planning. You have complete freedom to do as you please (your spouse?) You benefit from all that you do or you take consequences for anything you do wrong. This is the ideal for those personalities who prefer to be independent, to make their own decisions and not have to face compromises (or losses).

Partnership

There can be multiple partners in a group, but here the term is used to indicate two or three physicians working together. Your independence is gone, replaced in the best situations with camaraderie and compromises. Decisions are made jointly (or by prior arrangement). Purchases are a joint effort. Monies are divided on a pre-arranged schedule. Hours are decided by the group—usually there is an attempt to equalize the work. This kind of situation is ideal for those physicians who like to work together, can agree within a group and compromise when necessary (provided one of the partners does not try to dominate the others).

An important consideration: You should choose (or accept) your partner or partners as carefully as you would choose your wife. Their goals in practice (regarding income, free time, academics, growth and other items of your concern) must be compatible, for the most part, with your goals. Incompatibility in these areas bodes poorly for your success and happiness in practice.

Group

I have included here larger groups (4 or more). Everything here requires group action or group acquiescence. There are more differences within this group—so the choices become more selective.

Service

These are generally salaried positions, not earnings-driven jobs. Many good physicians choose to fill service positions—public health jobs, military positions, school health and the like. In this group, there are many variations; in some, the actual medical practice is dictated, and in some, not. Many good physicians prefer the controlled mode, with hours being set, salary potentials clear, and strong emphasis on service. Among most of these physicians, the honor of service over-rides all other aspects of choice.

Administrative

Some physicians prefer to become emergency room chiefs, clinic directors, company doctors and the like. These are salaried positions with less freedom in how one practices. In fact, many of such jobs are non-practice positions. Mostly, however, top jobs are not open to newly-minted graduates. It may be necessary to work your way up to be a "chief". If one of these positions is interesting to you, probably you should consider earning a Master of Business Administration degree, as many employers demand or request that of such employees

This has not been an attempt to define or categorize all the types of practice one can enter—merely a brief description (with many variations and overlaps) of the types of practice available.

In my own case, I went into another doctor's office, as an independent practitioner, and subsequently moved into my own offices, as these were only options open to me at that time (1946). Subsequently, I took on a partner (one whom I had trained) and it happened to be a most compatible team. I was totally satisfied with my situation and was a happy practitioner. It must have fit my personality.

The important thing for you, the reader, is to examine yourself, your likes and dislikes, consider your immediate family and be sure you do not pursue some practice that carries too many of your dislikes. Your happiness in your job is your most important consideration. Don't be confused by glamour or money!

Do you prefer to work alone, or with other people? Can you tolerate group decisions? Do you want someone to tell you what hours to work? Do you have the urge to serve? What will your spouse/family prefer in living arrangements? These and many other considerations that I have pointed out need to be taken into your thoughts—preferably before you start your search.

For some, making an actual written list of preferences might help your decision-making. but be sure that you include those things you dislike.

Who Will Be Your Patients? And What Will They Bring?

These are important questions in order for you to understand how to provide good patient care. Knowing who you are dealing with and what "baggage" they bring with them to your office will make it easier for you deliver outstanding service.

Who will be your patients?
Jump forward a few years and take a look into your waiting room. There's an auto mechanic, a nurse, a secretary, a major company executive, a plumber, a lawyer, an accountant, a mother, a father, a grandmother, a grandfather, a gambler, two people with arrest records, a process server, a detective—in other words, representatives from all walks of life.

You must be able to converse with all of them (even the deaf ones), maintain friendship and complete your medical activities in a friendly manner. Quite a task!

Some may have heavy accents. Some may be hard of hearing or have visual difficulties, some may have to be helped physically to get on your examining table or to walk, some may be very old and some very young. But you have to be prepared for a wide variety of people entering your office every day.

What will they bring?

For most, who they are will be less important than what they bring. Of course, they will all bring a medical complaint and with your training and background, you will probably be ready to face that.

But what is hidden may cause you problems and you are not likely to spend the time inquiring about them. Patients will come with some fright, anxiety, fear, anger, distrust, overconfidence—or all of these. Some will be concerned because they have never met you before. Some will, in the same situation, be afraid—of the outcomes, of their handling, of the costs. Some will be worried about a child they had to leave with a neighbor in order to visit you. Some will be upset because they had to take off work to keep your appointment.

So patients will come to you not just with a medical problem, but carrying the "baggage" of outside considerations—many times interfering with their "hearing" you, or understanding you or remembering the essentials of their visit. And you must be able to treat them through all that.

It is more than just your wading through your patients' problems; there may be some "baggage". If you discover it, maybe you can actually help the patient with it, or it may even be connected with the patient's complaints. Such discovery can create greater patient satisfaction and more acceptance of your therapy suggestions.

It is not a question of a fixed, stereotypical relationship for every person; all patients bring their own sets of cultures, their own background, and their own personal problems. Thus, it is urgent that you have excellent interpersonal relations with your patients. It will help their cooperation. It will help their acceptance of your ministrations. It will help their understanding. It will help their medical condition. And it will help you achieve greater success in your medical work!

Part Two

The Interpersonal Relationships

For ease of understanding, in this section, I will talk as though you have chosen to go into solo practice. Everything will be germane to one-doctor practice. If you are looking at other types of practice, this can serve as a template or pattern against which to measure the potential for you of any multi-doctor practice.

Your Office

Your office (you, your staff, your décor and furnishings) by its simple existence sends a message or messages to your patients—noisy, quiet, rude, patient-oriented, professional, or whatever). In general, it represents YOU and helps form your patient's impression of you.

As I have said, I will not discuss the business and management details of entering a practice, unless they bear upon the interpersonal relationships. Here are some that do just that.

Physical office

Your physical office will be with you for a long time, so putting it together (or evaluating an existing situation) requires advance good thinking. Décor is not the theme of this book. You should be looking for a set-up that is comfortable, pleasant to the eye and clean. Comfortable seating is more important than style or artistic themes. Comfort and cleanliness are the guiding principles.

Your staff

At some time in your practice, you will need staff to assist you. It may be one person or several, but these suggestions apply whichever it is.

In almost all cases, the staff is YOU. If you want them to be cordial, they will be cordial; if you allow them to be rude, they will be rude. Among the frequent complaints about doctor's staff people are rudeness, arrogance, indifference and the like. Conversely, there are many instances in which office staff is the key to patient satisfaction by developing splendid relations with patients. Remember, you have the power of hiring and firing, so if you tolerate poor behavior, they are a reflection on you. and patients will carry away that impression.

I have heard reports that occasional doctors say, "I know she's rude and hard to get along with, but she is such an outstanding bookkeeper (or clerk or secretary) that I can't let her go." Baloney! If she's alienating patients, making them unhappy with your office and sometimes losing them for you, it's better to fire her now and get the next-best bookkeeper (or whatever)! If you allow such activity to go on, it means that you want it that way or just don't care about patients and what they think. Neither reason will help you develop a practice.

Major question: Are your staff people friendly and helpful or are they rushed and arrogant? Remember that all behavior of your staff transmits messages to patients about your office . . . and YOU! Think about this—in advance

Staff must pay prompt attention to patients and their needs, be nice to them, call them by name, greet them kindly. And actually, it's easier to do that than to be perverse. It's your responsibility to train them and let them know exactly how you want patients treated.

Then, there's that little problem—the little window. You know, the window separating the waiting room from the office staff. Meant to be a place to greet patients, to help them with paper work and to inform them, so many times it is used by some staff as a barrier—to keep them disconnected from the patients (or "to keep them from annoying us"). I have often wondered what it is in the inner office that is so secretive that it has to be hidden from the patients in the waiting room. Whenever I've been privy to the inner workings, I saw nothing but office staff, desks, telephones—you know, a typical office. No wild parties or other forbidden activity. Why, then, cut off the patients and even keep them from asking questions or seeking help? If you really want to hide your office and office staff, there needs to be a re-arrangement of the partitions so that patients have ready access to the staff (or to a receptionist).

In hiring, or training, do not assume that previous employment is another doctor's office will suffice and be satisfactory for your office. That doctor may not practice the way you want to or seek the same results. Make sure your help does things the way you want them. You train them!

The telephone—boon or bane

Just for a moment, imagine what practice life would be like without the use of the telephone: Patients couldn't call you, the hospital could not reach you, you would not be able to order supplies in a hurry . . . and even personal items as talking to your spouse, getting a call from your child's school, notice of a repairman's visit. The list is endless.

Yes, the telephone was and is a marvelous invention and is being improved every day. It gives us service and help of infinite variety.

But, therein lurks also some dangers—not from the telephone itself but in the way that we use it.

Many times, it is the first connection with you. Does your staff answer with a hurried, half-hearted hello or, even worse, a "Yeah?" When you first taste a new food and it's awful, do you keep coming back for more in the hope that you might eventually like it? Hardly likely! One never gets a second chance to make a first impression, and first impressions are extremely important. So train your staff to greet all callers with a warm, friendly voice, with a cordial greeting and with an offer of service or a message, something like "Good morning, this is Dr. Brown's office. Can I help you?" Or "Is there something I can do for you?' There are a multitude of variants. But it must be warm, unhurried and convey some important message. If the office is closed and a voice on the machine answers, it should say—again, something like—"You've reached Dr. Brown's office. I'm sorry but the office is closed now. If you need . . ." (and finish out the message for what to do). End with "Thank you for calling us."

But I must congratulate you for having your staff answer instead of a recorded message center. I have yet to meet any person—not one—who likes to have several choices and has to live through a list of optional numbers to learn which "number to push." In many ways, it is cruel and saves very little time or money. Nothing connects like a human voice, and if it's a welcoming voice, you are halfway home with your opening. If you do use a system, do not have more than 2 or 3 choices; callers rebel at being given 6 or 8 choices. If the number of possible connections increases beyond the simple handling, there is all the more reason for a human voice to steer the caller—and save everybody's time.

A service greatly appreciated by patients (and others) is prompt answering of telephones and prompt call-back when required. A small mid-western businessman built a multi-million dollar enterprise, in part on his two rules: every incoming fax had to be replied to within 15 minutes and every phone call had to be answered by a human being within three rings. Promptness pays off.

Besides training your staff in the appropriate reception of calls, it is also necessary to train them in how you want them to handle many other matters—billings, complaints or other angry calls, threats, and the like. Old but true: A soft voice turneth away wrath. When that doesn't work, nothing will.

<u>Cell phones.</u> Modern developments have brought us another marvelous device that brings with it potential problems—the cell phone. The problems are on both sides of the telephone line.

Many doctors have been plagued by patients sitting in the waiting room and receiving or sending cell phone calls (or walking around the waiting room while talking). Sometimes it is because of a long wait for the appointment; sometime it is pure inconsideration of the user. If you haven't observed it, try to do so. Generally, patients are annoyed by listening to chats about grocery lists, last night's dinner, and so on . . . endlessly. Many physicians' offices have now banned use of cell phones in the office, or strongly requested that they not be used.

But what about the doctor? Aye, there's the rub! So many of us tend to ignore our own rules about cell phones as if they do not apply to us.

Mrs. N arrived on time for her appointment (another actual case). After a reasonably short wait, she was ushered into the examining room. The doctor came in, greeted her, spoke briefly with her and then started to examine her. His cell-phone rang! Saying excuse me to Mrs. N, he left the room . . . for about fifteen minutes. I presume that if it were about a dying patient or a patient who just arrived at the Emergency Department or something of that order, he would have apologized on his return and briefly explained the urgency of the call. What important message could it have been for someone to call on his personal line during office hours? Bring home a loaf of bread? Stop and get the tire fixed? Hey, doc, this is your broker calling? It could be any or all or others. But it was an annoyance to the patient and a big time delay for her and those patients who followed her.

Doctors usually have staff members who can pick up their calls, take a message and save it for the doctor—between patients or at the end of the day. For the just-mentioned patient, it was a black mark for the physician. A few more black marks and who knows what would happen. Cell phones can be important, but as long as someone can answer the office phone, the doctor should not use a cell phone in the office. An aide can interrupt, if the call is a matter of medical urgency or life and death.

Again, the telephone is a blessing but must be controlled—both physician and patients. Maybe a suggestive sign in the waiting room something like

I've turned off my cell-phone.
Won't you do likewise?

Patient's names

Our names are important to all of us, and we want to be identified by those names.

That also applies to patients.

One of the major national medical clinics instructs its personnel (all of them—nurses, doctors, aides, janitors) to greet every patient with "Good Morning, Mrs. James" or its equivalent (if they know the name) or just "Good Morning" (if they do not know the name). Patients talk about that, they often brag about it, they like it and they develop a stronger attachment to the group. The same certainly can be done in a smaller practice, without increased effort or cost or time. Why not develop satisfied customers . . . er, satisfied patients?

One question that always comes up is the use of first names. When uncertain, always use Mr., Mrs. or Ms. My easy rule is to use a first name only if you are otherwise acquainted on a first name basis; if not, use the formal title. Remember our customs say that if someone calls you by your first name, you have a right to return in kind. So, if you call Mr. Cordes "George", don't be surprised if he starts to calls you "Tom". I believe (and some may differ), that such formality does belong in the doctor's office. I always used Mr. or Mrs. for my patient's parents, except when they were personal friends or I had some other good reason to be informal. Start with the formal; it's always easier to go from that to first name than to go in the other direction.

Another suggestion for making patients more comfortable in the office is to have readily visible name tags for staff, with first names large (and, optionally, last names in smaller type). But use printed tags for the staff, not raggedy hand-written ones. That also makes it easier for a patient to identify a staff person by being able to say "Joanne" instead of "That blond girl out there with one earring and wearing a blue dress."

Appointments

Probably the most frequent complaint about doctors' offices is the appointment problem. And most of these complaints revolve around patients having to wait long beyond their appointed time. The problem is widespread and is alleviated or remedied only with concentrated effort and time. There is no perfect solution but like any other on-going difficulty efforts to correct it should be on-going also. Perhaps in its entirety it is an insoluble problem but continual attention to it can probably produce improved conditions. The operative word is "continual"—very few appointment programs are good and workable for ever.

Why is there such a problem? It can be attributed to either the doctor's (or his/her staff's) realm or to something on the patient's side. Mainly the patient's side is the existence of new symptoms or problems with established therapy requiring added attention and time. There are a great number of variables but since we are talking about doctors, we will address that side here. In none of this is blame being leveled.

Several reasons are in the doctor's purview. Do we really know in advance how to set up a patient schedule—or do we rely on a strict clock schedule—15 minutes, 20 minutes, 30 minutes—without regard to what those visits constitute? Do we allow the appropriate increased time for new patients? (New patients always require much more time and should be so scheduled). Do we actually know how much time we take with an average new patient? Do we sometimes "squeeze" in an extra patient, delaying all patients after that? Or do we sometimes double-book (to avoid "dead space" in our work)? Perhaps a few physicians just don't care. ("I'm the doctor and I'm a very busy person. Let them wait for me.")

At a social gathering I attended, a physician loudly bragged, "When I get to the office at 9 in the morning, there already are a dozen patients waiting for me." Questioned why he did not set up appointments, he answered, "Oh, no. This way the patients are impressed with what a good doctor I must be." No comment necessary!

Not caring is unacceptable. There can be occasional incidents forcing a delay (through no fault of the physician) and that's understandable—notice that I said "occasional". If they are regular, they should be able to be built into your schedule. And you must stay aware of such occurrences in your office and try to minimize them. The occasional one can be ameliorated by a brief explanation to the patient at the time with an apology and most patients would excuse it.

We must realize that in most offices, staff members make the appointments, so the doctor is not always involved—but he or she is always responsible. Not long ago, I called a very busy executive for an appointment (not medical but at least as busy). The first question from the secretary was, "About how much time will you need with him?" Great question—showing obvious concern for the caller while protecting the executive's schedule. Comparably, what would be wrong or difficult if a physician's appointment staff asked something like these questions: "Are you a new patient?" or for re-visits, "Do you have anything new to tell the doctor—new complaint, new symptom—or is this just a check-up visit?"

To the best of one's ability, appointments should be based on what procedures and medical care have to be provided at each visit and each doctor's average timing for all of them. Difficult to do, but rewarding in the attempt.

I made a second appointment with a doctor whom I had visited once before—and unfortunately at that time, I was seen 1 1/2 hours after the appointed time. I gave him the benefit of the doubt and returned. This next visit, I was kept in the waiting room for 90 minutes, then placed in an examination room. I waited there, unseen, for another half-hour, two hours waiting time. I stormed out and wrote the doctor what I thought: simply that he did not know how to book patients . . . or didn't care. *Repeated* latenesses are not from pressures of practice but are due to indifference.

Here is the spot for a practice management consultant, and there are many good ones around. This is one of their specialties. While I am not privy to their methods and work, I suspect it's something like this. They evaluate the kinds (and percentages) of certain visits and procedures and the doctor's time required for each one, then arrange a schedule of appointments that will help the doctor to keep his appointments (and still be able to predict when he will be finished.).

Let's hypothesize (and over-simplify). Say you take one hour (some practitioners may take more or less) for a new patient visit. And for a routine re-visit, 15 minutes. The consultant's survey shows you have an average of one new patient a day. So, he allows a full-hour space once each day, and the rest of the patients will be on time. Caveat: Do not use that one-hour space to "squeeze in" another patient. "But . . . but . . . ," I can hear you sputtering, "what if that hour-long appointment is cancelled or the patient doesn't show up?" Good, legitimate question. If cancelled early enough, fill the space with last-minute requests for appointment, or if it's a late cancellation or a "no-show", here's your opportunity to play catch-up, to do some of that painful paper work, to call-back certain patients waiting to hear from you, to check with the hospital on some condition of one of your patients (all things you would have to do later). You will always find something important to fill the time. And if it's a frequent occurrence, it can be built into your schedule.

What do I consider a reasonable wait for an appointment in a physician's office? Arbitrarily, I think 15 or 20 minutes, with an outside of 30 minutes—except for that occasional "catastrophic" occurrence (which does happen from time to time). Remember that many physicians (in different specialties as well as family medicine) usually are able to maintain short waiting room times.

And speaking about waiting times raises the issue of length of time from the request for appointment to the assigned time. Mrs. L sought consultation with a specialist—a so-called super-specialist—and had to wait four weeks, while continuing to endure her chief complaint. You as a beginning physician will probably not run into such a volume of patients for a long time, but it is good to keep in mind that this does occur in medical practice—and everyone should try to minimize it.

You, the doctor

While all the other things we discuss are important, the most important is YOU—in providing medical care, in pleasing patients, in meeting their needs and in making it inviting for them to come back when needed.

<u>The first visit.</u> Assuming that a staff member has placed the patient in an examining or consultation room, you will want to greet the patient by name (partially to make a personal connection and partly to make sure it is the right patient), then introduce yourself, so the patient knows that you are the right doctor (especially if several doctors practice at the same location). For example, "Hello, Mr. Visker, I'm Dr. Greene" or "Good Afternoon, Mr. Visker. I'm Dr. Greene". Allowing a brief moment for the patient's reply, you must then offer your lead question—why the patient is here. "How can I help you?" Or "What can I do for you today?"

Because many times patients have more than one question or anxiety, one physician suggested "And what two things can I help you with today?" That does not limit the patient to a single item and allows for more than one topic. (Many times, the two or three problems are related and immediately help with the diagnosis.)

On follow-up visits, you should use the greeting, but not necessarily giving your name, and using a follow-up question: "Hello, Mrs. Visker. What can I help you with today?" or "Hi, Mrs. Visker, did the medication help you? How are you feeling now?"

It probably adds some warmth to your visits if your repeat her name each visit—but you have to use your judgment. Following this pattern, you can use your own wording in your own style. (But not like the physician quoted earlier who said, "Don't talk to me.")

<u>Listen to the Patient.</u> Still one of the soundest bits of advice is the aphorism of Osler—"Listen! The patient is telling you the diagnosis" Meant to stress the importance of the medical history, it also applies to creating a workable, or even great, interpersonal relationship. True, some patients will be reticent and you have to drag information out of them and some will be so verbose that you almost cannot stop them. But somewhere between is the patient's history (and an expose of his/her personality). Most important is that when you listen, the patient gets the impression of a kindly, interested doctor.

<u>Body Language.</u> A little more esoteric than much of these suggestions, it is still something worthwhile—a consideration for both you and the patient Body language is said, by various sources, to make up 60% to 90% of interpersonal communication. Body language includes eyes and eye movements, facial expressions, body positions and leg and arm movements. So it would be helpful if you learn at least a few of the body signs, so that you understand the patient better and so that you

do not give any negative signals (sometimes patients recognize body language without being conscious of it). Some common ones of import, for example, are:

> Eye contact—shows interest and concentration
> Arms folded across chest—resistance to what is being said or done
> Twiddling of fingers or feet—boredom, indifference
> Extended arm and hand (at least 3 seconds)—gesture of friendliness
> Hand to cheek—evaluation, thinking
> Tilted head—interest

These are just a few examples of body language. Some you will learn by experience. Others, if you have time to study them, will make you appear more interested or avoid seeming negative to patients—and, in turn, you will be able to interpret patient's communication from their body language.

And what about <u>your</u> non-verbal communication? Do you, unconsciously, send certain signals to patients? Are they negative? Can you improve on this? It's worth a little study on your part.

<u>Dress</u>. Who? What? The physician should always be neatly dressed, not ostentatious or sloppy. I believe that the doctor on duty should wear a tie and jacket with or without a white coat (long or short). A few contend that a little more informality is satisfactory—no tie, or no jacket—but certainly not a short sleeve sport shirt. Judging the patient is a bit harder: Is he overdressed (trying to impress you), sloppy (is this his personality?).

I have heard tales of well-to-do people dressing down to impress the doctor with being poor. A number of years ago, a major Philadelphia hospital did a survey of its patients—just at the time when residents were taking to wearing Jeans, or sport shirts, or sandals. The surprising result was that patients were satisfied and not upset at the residents' dress, but, please note, they wanted their attending physicians to be dressed in tie and jacket.

Comparable suggestions apply to female physicians. Very often, patients will seek out doctors who dress as they expect them to—usually more formally; they do believe that a direct relationship exists between dress and skills.

Ending a visit. Sounds like there's nothing to it, eh? Not at all. A New England Journal of Medicine study of a large number of Medicare patients in several different hospitals revealed that 20% of Medicare patients are readmitted within 30 days. From that study, there developed a program of improving discharge procedures for hospitals. (I can personally testify, after experiencing a number of hospital discharges, that most of the time it is an abominable procedure—totally inadequate.) That program was called Project RED (Re-Engineered Discharge). Then, 30 hospitals installed a Project RED, with marked success, greatly reducing the number of re-admissions and proving the thesis correct. It consists of 11 specific discharge steps.

Reasoning from that to the office, transforming office discharge procedures might also eliminate or reduce unnecessary re-visits, thus providing better care for patients. Give serious consideration to formal patient instructions (other than a clerk saying "Mrs. Crow, you don't have to come back any more!" or "Mrs. Crow, call your doctor in a week and take this prescription" (handing the patient the prescription without further information). It should include medication instructions, any other health matters, when to return, phone calls from your office if the patient does not keep the appointment, and similar follow-ups.

This visit is the time for summarizing the medical aspects, whether end of visit or on discharge. Everything should be explained clearly with no jargon in your attempt to be sure the patient understands

One of the most important items in a discharge visit—or any other visit—is asking the question "Do you have any questions?" So often, patients still have unspoken or unsolved questions that they don't get a chance to ask. I believe that no interview should ever be ended without that question. An additional factor is that the question sends a hidden message: I am not rushing you and I am interested in you." You might even find more reason to treat or uncover more pathology. At least, you will have a patient walk away satisfied.

Your Writings

This worthwhile subject is included because it is almost never taught in our schools or training programs, and is an extremely important practical aspect of practice.

Two specific things that you will be writing in your professional activities deserve comment—comment intended to help you avoid problems. They are Letter Writing and Prescription Writing. You may or may not be writing letters early in your career but it is wise to consider the problems now.

Letter Writing

I presume, since all my readers will be college graduates, that you have a good idea about writing letters, so I will touch only on the parts and forms in which there may be a problem.

    Suggestions:
- Be sure to date every letter
- In the salutation, do not write "Dear Bob" unless you know Bob on a first name basis. Otherwise, always address the person by Mr., Mrs., Ms., Dr., Rev. (no degrees).
- Be sure your complimentary closing is appropriate, for example, do not use Respectfully if it is a nasty letter, and

do not use Cordially unless there is a cordial relationship.

Things to avoid:

"I would like to . . ." If you'd really like to, go ahead and say it. You do not have to introduce it.

"With best regards I am (or something similar). The use of "I am . . ." is old fashioned and should not be used.

"Dictated but not read" This is used by consultants who believe it exonerates them from any mistakes in the letter. Not so! But, more important, it says to the reader "I don't think enough of you or this letter to spend an infinitesimal amount of time checking it or signing it." Very inconsiderate! Plus, there could be mistakes in dictation (some things sound alike) or mistakes in the secretary's transcription (Does anyone have a secretary who *never* makes a mistake? And *rarely* does not exonerate you.)

"I saw your interesting patient" Some consultants write this as part of a form letter. Do not start a consultation report with such a line. After the third letter of consultation from you, the referring doctor will realize it is pure bull and therefore worthless.

Having someone else sign the letter. (Or rubber-stamping your name.) Seems to send the same message as "Dictated . . ."

Signature:
In a professional letter, sign your name in full with proper identification. Dr. Jules Brach is an improper form for this; the signature should be Jules Brach, DO. By the way, your letterhead and envelope should read Jules Brach, DO, never Dr. Jules Brach. However, in a salutation, use "Dear Dr. Brach"

Prescription Writing

Most prescription blanks are sufficiently structured for an adequate fill-in. But there are some precautions. However, since the Institute of Medicine estimates that about 7,000 deaths a year occur because of prescription errors, we must be extra careful or extra. extra careful!

In 2003, the state of Florida, aiming to reduce prescription errors, passed a law that said that all prescriptions are required to:

be legibly printed or typed;

contain the name of the prescribing practitioner, the name and strength of the drug prescribed, the quantity of the drug prescribed in both textual and numerical formats, and the directions for the use of the drug;

be dated with the month written out in textual letters; and be signed by the prescribing practitioner on the day when issued.

Seeing that some of the prescriptions I received were incorrectly written, I gave several fine practitioners a copy of the new law. They thanked me but continued to write their Rx the same old way.

To those physicians just starting out, I say—strongly—start by keeping within the law. From then on, you will do it by habit. And maybe avoid going to jail or paying a huge fine (plus the embarrassment).

<u>Some suggestions</u>:
- Write clearly or print or type the Rx.
- Always include the age—it is helpful to the pharmacist.
- Include patient's weight—it may help evaluate the dosage, especially in children.
- Including the diagnosis might be helpful when the pharmacist cannot read the Rx.
  Don't worry about privacy, it's a communication between professionals about the same patient. The ordered drug will often give away the diagnosis.
- When giving a patient a prescription (and I advise that the doctor himself do it—no clerks or cashiers), hand it directly to the patient, say the drug out loud and then ask the patient to read the Rx back to you. It's great insurance—and it costs you no extra premium.

Rules?

(Not really, just recommendations for a successful practice)

A Summary

1. Train your staff in the ways you want them to act, and enforce it.
2. Be sure you and your staff realize the importance of telephone talk.
3. Eliminate cell-phones from your office (doctor and patients) as far as possible.
4. Be careful in the use of patients' first names.
5. Pay strict attention to your appointment schedule. Watch for times when there is long delay and fix it. Don't be afraid to revise your schedule from time to time.
6. Pay attention to letters you write. They reflect YOU.
7. Be extremely careful in writing prescriptions and transmitting them to patients.
8. Good patient interaction calls for:
    Being friendly at office visits—especially the first one
    Developing some interest in body language, both yours and your patients
    Being careful of your office dress
    Learning good methods for closing out office visits

Always keep in mind the two great aphorisms (sources unknown) that lead to successful practice

Patients are not dependent on us . . . we are dependent on them

and

**Patients are not an interruption of our work . . . they are the purpose of it.
We are not doing our patients a favor by serving them
. . . they are doing us a favor by giving us the opportunity to do so**

**And
Good
Luck!!!**

www.ingramcontent.com/pod-product-compliance
Lightning Source LLC
Chambersburg PA
CBHW021026180526
45163CB00005B/2137